Alkaline I

Blast Fat, Lose Weight with the Alkaline Diet

Nicole Harrington

Gamma Mouse
www.gammamouse.com

ALKALINE DIET FOR BEGINNERS
Copyright © 2014 by Nicole Harrington.
All rights reserved.

First Edition: September 2014
1234567890
A Gamma Mouse eBook
Published by Gamma Mouse, a dba of Xilytics, LLC.
www.gammamouse.com

This document is geared towards providing exact and reliable information in regards to the topic and issue covered. The publication is sold with the idea that the publisher is not required to render accounting, officially permitted, or otherwise, qualified services. If advice is necessary, legal or professional, a practiced individual in the profession should be ordered.

From a Declaration of Principles which was accepted and approved equally by a Committee of the American Bar Association and a Committee of Publishers and Associations.

In no way is it legal to reproduce, duplicate, or transmit any part of this document in either electronic means or in printed format. Recording of this publication is strictly prohibited and any storage of this document is not allowed unless with written permission from the publisher. All rights reserved.

The information provided herein is stated to be truthful and consistent, in that any liability, in terms of inattention or otherwise, by any usage or abuse of any policies, processes, or directions contained within is the solitary and utter responsibility of the recipient reader. Under no circumstances will any legal responsibility or blame be held against the publisher for any reparation, damages, or monetary loss due to the information herein, either directly or indirectly.

Respective authors own all copyrights not held by the publisher.

The information herein is offered for informational purposes solely, and is universal as so. The presentation of the information is without contract or any type of guarantee assurance.

The trademarks that are used are without any consent, and the publication of the trademark is without permission or backing by the trademark owner. All trademarks and brands within this book are for clarifying purposes only and are the owned by the owners themselves, not affiliated with this document.

Introduction

Helping people lose weight has become a huge part of my life. And being able to teach other people the knowledge I have gained has become extremely important to me.

I consider my readers my friends. I am always so appreciative that they take the time out to read my books and to learn about various diets from me.

Once you have finished with this book, I have no doubt that you will have learned a great deal about how to get the results you are looking for. You will be on the first step to really living the life you have always desired.

With just a little effort and the right information, you will be amazed at what you can accomplish.

Let's get started!

Limited Time Free Offer

Download the #1 Bestseller from Gamma Mouse Media for FREE! Hurry this offer won't last as it is for a limited time only. Reserve your free copy today at http://gammamouse.com.

The Alkaline Diet – What It Can Do for You

In recent years, one diet plan has been gaining a steady stream of popularity and renown: the alkaline diet. What the diet purports to do sounds wonderful: it helps you lose weight, it can increase your overall energy. It also has laid claim to being able to lessen one's anxiety, eliminate headaches, and even combat the common cold and flu.

These type of claims are easy to make, but does the Alkaline diet live up to its tremendous hype, can it really do what it claims it does? Early results have been promising, but to understand more about this diet we need to take a closer look first.

The Science behind the Alkaline Diet

The human body is a remarkably efficient machine, always maintaining a balance. When things get out of balance is when problems can occur. This equilibrium state of the body is also known as homeostasis. One of the most obvious examples is when we perspire when we workout, the body is naturally attempting to cool itself down. This same concept applies to opposite end of the spectrum, when we shiver when it is cold outside.

One of the measurements of homeostasis in the body is referred to as pH, which measures the alkalinity of the body. We don't want to get too scientific, so let's just understand that pH is represented on a scale from 1 to 14, with the higher number being more alkaline. Normally, the blood wants a pH level of around 7.5. Anything outside of this area is a definite cause of concern as it means that your body is not working both efficiently and properly. This can obviously have significant repercussions on your health.

What is the pH of Food?

When you eat a meal, your body goes through the process of digestion, absorbing the nutrients of the food into the bloodstream. All of these foods that we eat end up releasing various compounds into our blood. These compounds could be alkaline, or they could be acidic. Foods are then separated in the alkaline scheme by whether they are considered to be acidic in nature or alkaline. Generally, dairy, meat and fish, sugar and grains are thought of as acidic. Vegetables and fruits as well as nuts and beans are typically alkaline. What we need to understand is that all foods release compounds into the blood which will affect your body's pH level. It sound appear clear that we will want to eat foods that maintain our optimal pH level.

The Alkaline Diet

The alkaline diet operates under this conceptual framework, assuming that overconsumption of acidic foods will cause our blood pH to fluctuate out of the optimal range, which in turn could cause our bodies to run less efficiently. Because the body strives for homeostasis, it will attempt to restore a slightly alkaline pH level. However during this time when our bodies are not working efficiently, we may be losing out on valuable nutrients. The theory behind this is that our body will be starved for nutrients and overconsumption could occur leading to gaining weight. A susceptibility to illnesses because of a weakened immune system is also possible.

Operating under this theory, the alkaline diet suggests a diet that matches the pH of our blood, this way we can maintain homeostasis and keep our bodies running smoothly and efficiently. This means that the alkaline diet encourages eating fresh vegetables and fruits as well as beans, tofu and nuts as sources of protein. These foods help to maintain the proper pH value. Foods that are to be avoided on the alkaline diet are sugar, grains, dairy and meat. Processed foods are also not permitted on the alkaline diet. Caffeine and alcohol are generally not allowed on the diet, however if you do wish to indulge, keep it limited to wine, coffee or tea.

Will It Work for You?

As you would expect for any recent diet, the final word on whether the diet will actually help you lose weight is still open to scientific debate. Unfortunately, the alkaline diet is just too new to have enough research behind for or against it. However, if one looks at the diet with eye towards what we do understand as being beneficial to losing weight—namely eating fruits and vegetables, avoiding grains and processed foods—the alkaline diet appears to be operating on a solid foundation. As with starting any new diet plan, it is always good to have a checkup and consultation with your medical provider who can go over the risks and benefits of your eating plan.

While the alkaline diet emphasizes healthy eating, certain individuals may not get enough vital nutrients if they strictly follow the diet. Eliminating meat for one's diet makes it more difficult to maintain proper levels of protein and iron. It should also be noted, that because you are interested in your pH level, you may want to set up regular testing in order to monitor it. Once again your doctor can help you with this.

The Benefits of the Alkaline Diet

Now that we have a basic understanding of the theory behind the alkaline diet, we can take a closer look at some of the diet's benefits. The main goal of the alkaline diet is to eat foods that will maintain the body's equilibrium. Proponents of the diet suggest that this will lead to better health and potentially weight loss. Additional benefits are an increase in energy level and the reduction, or even elimination, of physical ailments that may plague us.

I like to think of the alkaline diet like a chemistry experiment. If we imagine our body as a test tube, it is important to understand and record what we put into that test tube. The point is that the alkaline diet requires a decent level of recording what we eat and seeing how that affects us. In an ideal setting, we would want to be able to monitor our pH level in order to make certain it stays within the optimal range. Each of our individual body chemistries can vary, thereby causing different reactions. This is where the chemistry comes into play; how you react and respond to a certain food may be entirely different than someone else.

Therefore, it is important that we try our best to monitor our pH level. While one could only eat the suggested foods and avoid the forbidden ones, this is not a guarantee of success if we have no clue of our pH level and how they are being affected by the different food components.

Alkaline Foods – Taking a Closer Look

To use a different metaphor, the foods we eat in the alkaline diet serve as a type of solution, either acidic in nature or alkaline. Our goal is to balance these foods in a way that we hit our optimum pH level of around 7.5. But the question then becomes what is the best way to hit this target.

At the most basic level, the alkaline diet suggests that you should avoid processed foods in favor or natural, organic foods like vegetables and fruits. For some people to lose weight, cutting out processed foods may be enough without having to go to further extremes by cutting out additional groups like meat and dairy. Others may require a much more delicate balancing act in which a limited selection of foods can be eaten. It is this group which needs to be consistently monitoring their pH level for fluctuations.

By avoiding certain food groups like meat and dairy, you are also depriving your body of specific nutrient sources. In this case, there could always be need to take a supplement in order to make certain that your body is getting all its required nutrients. If you have a vitamin or mineral imbalance that could definitely affect your results even if your pH level is in the acceptable range.

The alkaline diet is really a diet in which you need to think and approach it like a scientist, which means testing and recording the response. Operating blindly might only not get you the results you desire, it could be causing you harm. This is why monitoring your food intake and how it affects you is incredibly important.

Why People Prefer the Alkaline Diet

If you are the type of person who always seems to be nursing a cold, congestion or flu, or you feel like you have a low energy level, you may be a great candidate for the alkaline diet. In the past, doctors have also suggested the diet for chronic headache sufferers or those with benign breast cysts among others.

The theory is that higher acidity levels affect the body's ability to deal with illness. Therefore, the suggestions is that lower one's acidity level will help boost the immune system which can then fight off any chronic problems the individual may be suffering from. One of the ways that you see this in practices is people reducing the amount of sodium in their diets, since salt is considered acidic. By reducing sodium, the hope is that your immune system will bounce back.

Studies have also shown that alkaline foods may help in preventing calcium-based kidney stones and may also help reduce the loss of muscle that comes with the onset of older age. Other studies have theorized that acidic foods may actually be harmful to our liver and kidneys, since they were not designed to filter out so many acidic components. It should also be clear that acidic foods could have the potential of leading to a risk for diabetes.

None of this should be a surprise. An emphasis on healthy natural foods as opposed to processed additive enriched foods would logically lead to these results. The alkaline diet should not be viewed as revolutionary, rather it is offering a scientific basis for ideas that are generally well-accepted in the realm of diet and nutrition. It has long been know that whole natural foods like fruits and vegetables are better for you than processed foods, because our bodies have been engineered by nature to respond best to whole unprocessed foods. The alkaline diet is about accepting your natural state and eating foods designed for your body. No gimmicks, just basic nutrition.

Where the alkaline diet appeals to people is the level of control and detail one can take in their diet. By measuring one's pH level you are able to quantify your diet, tweaking here and there until you get the right combination. So fundamentally the alkaline diet is a very personal diet, specific to you.

Learning to Live the Alkaline Way

Whenever a new diet comes along, people always have the same question: why is this diet any different from the other diets? What makes it different from the liquid diets, low carb diets, crash diets, and detox diets?

At this point, the answer should be obvious: those diets are only concerned with the number that shows up when you step on the scale. The alkaline diet is not focused on weight as the measurement of success or failure, rather the measurable in the alkaline diet is an individual's pH level.

It is very important to understand that the alkaline diet is not focused solely on weight loss. That is only a potential consequence of monitoring you pH level and assuring that it maintains an optimal level. Weight loss is a benefit as is improved health and increased energy. The goal for the alkaline dieter is to focus on maintaining the proper pH level and not judging their success or failure by what the scale says.

Weight Loss

Since the goal of the alkaline diet is not weight loss, why should dieters who want to lose weight try the alkaline diet? Simply, the diet demands that you eat right. It demands that you avoid high carbohydrate, additive-enriched foods. It isn't a secret that most processed food has a higher calorie content than natural foods like fruits and vegetables. Eating less calories is almost natural when you start the alkaline diet, because it is hard to eat a comparable amount of calories if your primary eating source are vegetables and fruits. People find it difficult often to eat enough calories from fruits and vegetables to even hit their resting metabolic rate.

The dietary restrictions of the alkaline diet are stricter than the majority of diets; this is another reason for the success of many of the alkaline dieters. It is a diet that lends itself to proper eating habits.

Improving Digestion

If you suffer from any type of digestion problems, the alkaline diet is a wonderful choice. It has helped many people combat digestive maladies like acid reflux, ulcers and gastritis. Part of its effectiveness is from the stringent monitoring of the individual's pH level, but also the food restrictions make the diet incredibly easy on the digestive system. Fiber is plentiful in the diet, which helps along digestion.

If you are the type of person who eats a lot of processed foods or red meat and find you have issues or digestion discomfort, I recommend trying the alkaline diet. Eliminating your current foods for fruits and vegetables could produce immediate and impactful results. And this is an easier solution than other pharmacological or medical solutions.

Chronic Diseases

Every day a new medical study seems to be published about a certain food leading to a chronic health problem. It is easy to get the inclination that no matter what we eat, we are doomed to be eating something that is killing us. The reason that the alkaline diet may be successful in hindering potentially chronic health problems like diabetes, cancer, and heart disease is the insistence on mainly eating produce. By relying on natural products, we are able to avoid many of the additives in processed food that could be leading to major health problems.

Once again, though, this is a side benefit of the diet. There is also the possibility that maintaining an optimal pH level could reduce the chance of suffering from heart disease, cancer or diabetes. The point is that the alkaline diet could reduce these health risks either through maintaining homeostasis or through proper diet.

Prevention of cancer

Just a side note in relation to cancer and the alkaline diet. Studies have shown that when a body has an acidic pH level, cellular metabolism could be hindered. This can lead to cancerous cells developing as a result. This of course is separate from cancer that could develop from dietary factors.

Boosting the Immunity System

Research has speculated that when the body's pH is in a state of imbalance it lends itself to being a perfect environment for infections and common illnesses since a higher acid level can lead to the immune system being compromised. A big reason for this is that at a cellular level when things are not operating under optimal conditions, it is much easier for foreign bodies to spread, causing infection and other illnesses caused by free-roaming bacteria and viruses. This has a tendency to tax the immune system.

The theory suggests, then, that by maintaining an optimal pH level, the body will be less hospitable to bacteria. This means that the immune system will be less taxed—and therefore more robust—since it is no longer fighter off constant threats of infection.

Increased Levels of Energy

We all want to feel great, to have enough energy to chance our kids or grandchildren around. But if our cells are not living in a healthy, balanced environment, they will be not only subject to possible infection, but they will no longer be transporting oxygen through the blood efficiently. This of course leads to feelings of tiredness and general malaise. Cellular ATP production is also affected when the pH conditions are less than ideal, which also has a dramatic impact on one's energy levels.

Hopefully you now have a better grip on the tremendous impact that the alkaline diet can have on your life. Not only does the alkaline diet have intended consequences that arise from maintaining an optimal pH level like, for example, cancer prevention. The diet could also have many side positive consequences that arises from such a restrictive diet. These would include potentially weight loss, boosting the immune system, and increasing energy levels. This is the major reason why I like to consider the alkaline diet a dual stream diet providing a multitude of potential health benefits.

What Not to Eat on the Alkaline Diet

The human body needs protein; it is essential to proper functioning. Research shows that protein that derives from animals releases acids like uric, sulfuric and phosphoric acid during digestion and absorption. Our kidneys are tasked with removing these acid products from our bloodstream. If meat is consumed in moderation, the kidneys have no problems dealing with filtering the blood, but excessive meat consumption and eventual breakdown will lead to the kidneys being overwhelmed in which case the acids will be stored in the body's tissue.

A vegetarian diet is not for everyone. The body still demands protein and meat offers a simple fix for this demand. At the very least, one should decrease their consumption of both meat and seafood when attempting the alkaline diet.

It is also recommended that all dairy products like butter, cheese, and milk be eliminated from your diet. One needs to recognize that much needed calcium will need to come from other sources. Iron and calcium supplements as well as a multivitamin will help to make up for the lack of dairy and meat products in one's diet.

All grains and rice are to be eliminated. Sugar and any foods with sugar type additives, like corn syrup, are also not allowed. Obviously, any type of fast food will land on this list. It is also encouraged that one limits their intake of sodium, too.

The alkaline diet is a highly restrictive diet. It can be difficult to implement, because it is a significant dietary change for most people. This is why I stress knowing your one measurable: your pH level. You may discover that you do not need to have such a restrictive diet in order to maintain an optimal level. Other individuals may have a much harder time. Once again, the alkaline diet is not a one-size-fits-all type of diet. The way your body responds to food will vary from someone else. This is why it is important to always keep your eye on your pH value.

What to Eat on the Alkaline Diet

Unfortunately, the foods allowed on the alkaline diet is a much smaller list than the foods that are disallowed.

For fruits and vegetables, there is no limit to what you are encouraged to eat on the alkaline diet. There is no need to only focus on green, leafy vegetables like broccoli, celery, and spinach. Other vegetables like cauliflower, carrots, and onions are just as important in the alkaline diet. A wide range of vegetables and fruits is encouraged in order to get the widest possible range of nutrients for your body.

One of the biggest difficulties on the alkaline diet is protein replacement. One of the major sources for protein is tofu. Other sources are healthy nuts like almonds as well as beans. Asian inspired dishes work well on the alkaline diet as long as you avoid most sauces. I suggest using lime or lemon juice to flavor your protein and vegetables. If you aren't familiar with cooking with a wok, I recommend learning; I have found it to be invaluable as an alkaline diet cooking method.

You can also flavor your food with cinnamon, curry and chili pepper, since all of these have alkaline properties. Because most of our modern food has high levels of salt, many people new to the diet find the food bland. My only suggestion is to experiment with different seasonings and natural juices. Sometimes throwing a citrus fruit into a savory dish can really help with bringing forth the full flavor of the dish.

The Alkaline Diet Starts With You

Make no mistake, starting the alkaline diet is a hard process. It will test you unlike most other diets. The key is to always be looking at the right number: your pH level and not the number on the scale. You may find that just by making small tweaks to your diet, you are able to obtain your optimal pH level. If that is the case, there is no reason to become more restrictive with the foods that you eat.

Realize that there are always people that will believe in you, that know that you can do it. Progress can be slow, hard even, but it is always being made even if you don't see it. Never give up! And always—always—keep your eye on the prize: an optimal pH level and a healthier you!

I wish you the best of luck!

WAIT! Before You Leave…

Download the #1 Bestseller from Gamma Mouse Media for FREE! Hurry this offer won't last as it is for a limited time only. Reserve your free copy today at http://gammamouse.com.

A Special Gift for Our Readers!

Thank you so much for your purchase of this book. As a special gift for you we have included one of our bestselling Self-Improvement books: Procrastination: Triple Your Productivity and Accomplish Your Goals written by one of the most well-respected and influential experts on time management, Warren R. Sullivan.

I hope you enjoy!

Procrastination
Triple Your Productivity and Accomplish Your Goals

Warren R. Sullivan

Gamma Mouse
www.gammamouse.com

PROCRASTINATION
Copyright © 2014 by Warren R. Sullivan.
All rights reserved.

First Edition: April 2014
1234567890
A Gamma Mouse eBook
Published by Gamma Mouse, a dba of Xilytics, LLC.
www.gammamouse.com

This document is geared towards providing exact and reliable information in regards to the topic and issue covered. The publication is sold with the idea that the publisher is not required to render accounting, officially permitted, or otherwise, qualified services. If advice is necessary, legal or professional, a practiced individual in the profession should be ordered.

From a Declaration of Principles which was accepted and approved equally by a Committee of the American Bar Association and a Committee of Publishers and Associations.

In no way is it legal to reproduce, duplicate, or transmit any part of this document in either electronic means or in printed format. Recording of this publication is strictly prohibited and any storage of this document is not allowed unless with written permission from the publisher. All rights reserved.

The information provided herein is stated to be truthful and consistent, in that any liability, in terms of inattention or otherwise, by any usage or abuse of any policies, processes, or directions contained within is the solitary and utter responsibility of the recipient reader. Under no circumstances will any legal responsibility or blame be held against the publisher for any reparation, damages, or monetary loss due to the information herein, either directly or indirectly.

Respective authors own all copyrights not held by the publisher.

The information herein is offered for informational purposes solely, and is universal as so. The presentation of the information is without contract or any type of guarantee assurance.

The trademarks that are used are without any consent, and the publication of the trademark is without permission or backing by the trademark owner. All trademarks and brands within this book are for clarifying purposes only and are the owned by the owners themselves, not affiliated with this document.

Introduction

Procrastination. It has a drastic effect on productivity, on our ability to accomplish our goals in life. It can greatly impact our happiness, as we avoid doing something that we are dreading. Yet having to do it still hangs over our head.

Delaying something in order to often do something easier is an easy trap to fall into. Do it enough, and it suddenly becomes a habit. The problem with procrastination is we usually put off more important—but also more difficult—objectives for doing actions that are more trivial. For example, a college student might watch television rather than write a report.

Our time is valuable. It is the one thing that cannot be replaced, unlike money or objects. Yet it is wasted when we procrastinate. Saving this time should be our goal. We need to realize that our time would be better spend on accomplishing our most important objectives. When you have finished those, then reward yourself.

Stopping our procrastination is as easy as changing our attitude and stopping the habit that we have fallen into. In reading this guide, you will learn the tips and tricks necessary to stop procrastinating and start living. You don't have to suffer any longer, you can be happy and more productive, accomplishing all the important goals in your life quickly and easily. But you must take the first step and make a commitment to change yourself. Reading this book is a start, but if you don't act on what you learn change will not come. So consider this a call to action, a chance to truly change your life.

Getting to the root of the problem

Everyone procrastinates. It is part of being human. Whether because of laziness or not having the energy to tackle a difficult task, we choose to relax, to take the easy way out. Understand that not all procrastination should be viewed as bad. Often we need a break from the rigors of our day, a chance to get away from the stress of life. Some goals require great effort and energy to complete, so tackling them when you don't have much energy is realistic.

The line we don't want to cross is when we fool ourselves into believing that laziness is not having the energy to complete our task. Our first step is to recognize when we are being lazy. Clearly, we need to be honest with ourselves, we need to hold ourselves accountable. Secondly, we need to realize that time is our most valuable resource, and that it is finite. No one knows how much time they have, so it is essential to understand how important time is. When you sit down to watch television, recognize that this is time you will never get back.

To borrow a phrase from economics, understand that there is an opportunity cost to ever action you take. When you choose to do something, you lose the opportunity to use that time differently. When you make a choice, there is always a cost, remind yourself of this when you find yourself procrastinating. One of my methods for reminding myself to utilize every minute of my time as effectively as I can is to write the number 1440 on the white board in my office. This is the number of minutes in one day. Whenever I find myself procrastinating, I look at my board, and it helps me refocus on my task at hand.

People procrastinate for different reasons. The first step is to understand the reasoning behind our procrastinating. There may be more than one, but understanding the psychology behind our choices will help us effectively combat them, allowing us to change our faulty reasoning when it arises.

Cognitive distortions are a form of irrational thinking that often lead to procrastination. It is a magically type of thinking. Often we believe that we will be better equipped at some point in the future to handle our task, rather than completely the task at that time.

An example is a person who believes that they need to be in a certain mood in order to complete a task successfully. Or a person may believe that their motivation will increase in the future, and thus will be in a better position to accomplish their goals. Another one that happens in business quite frequently is an employee overestimating the time they have left to complete a task while also underestimating how long it will take them to do it.

If you are putting off a task, because you believe that you will be better suited in the future, realize that you are committing a fallacy. There is no evidence suggesting that your belief is true.

When we are confused about how to complete a task, and the details involved, we may procrastinate giving the reason that we need further instructions before we can continue. This allows us to set the project aside, until we find that we are butting up against a deadline. This reasoning often comes up with perfectionists who do not want to start a task until they are confident in their ability to complete it perfectly. To combat this reasoning, understand that completely the task initially to the best of your abilities and understanding, and then waiting for feedback is much more productive. It is easy to make corrections to your mistakes once the task is completed, as opposed to trying to do the task perfectly the first time. And there is always the possibility that the goal will be accomplished on your first attempt, without the need for further clarification. Don't fool yourself into thinking that if you have additional information, you will be better suited to complete the task. This is a cognitive distortion.

An offshoot of this is avoiding a task because you don't know how it should be done, that you require procedural information. Once again, this reasoning arises most often in the perfectionist, who believes they need to wait for the perfect situation in order to be successful. But look at the great inventors throughout history, who only through trial and error found out how to accomplish something amazing. Imagine if they had waited for the perfect moment, these inventions may never have come into existence. Remember that your goal is to accomplish your task, mistakes that you make can always be corrected. Don't fear failure. Instead, recognize it as an opportunity to learn.

I used to suffer from thinking I needed to take the time, to contemplate and reflect, before beginning a job. What I was doing was procrastinating, convincing myself I needed more information. This was clearly a logical fallacy. Thinking about the job was not going to make me more productive. What was going to make me more productive was doing it. If you believe you need more time to accomplish something, stop and examine whether that is true. Even if it is true, you can start the task now and revise it later as your thoughts begin to coalesce.

    We have all had tasks that we had to do that we really didn't want to do. Income taxes come to mind. It is a responsibility, and sometimes that additional pressure makes a task unpleasant. And we are human, we do not want to do things we find unpleasant. We may even fool ourselves into thinking that there will be a point in the future when it will be easier to deal with an unpleasant task. Never make the mistake to think that a task that is unpleasant today will somehow miraculously improve in the future. It is always better to get the unpleasantness over immediately, rather than wait. I am reminded of my public speaking class in college. I always wanted to go first, and I could never understand why people wouldn't want to be first. Most found public speaking uncomfortable and unpleasant, but instead of immediately getting it out of the way and then relaxing, they chose to prolong how long the task would take them. Don't fall victim to this. If you find a task unpleasant, do it immediately; procrastination only makes it worse, and in the process makes you unhappy.

Now the opposite of procrastinating over tasks that we find unpleasant is to procrastinate over accomplishing goals that we don't care about. Finding the effort to complete a task when you are indifferent to the outcome is difficult. Often we may believe that we will feel more inclined to complete a task in the future when we feel more connected with the outcome. Usually indifference does not change, people don't suddenly start to care. These types of tasks often don't get tackled until we run up against a deadline. This can cause us additional stress as we must now take time to complete a task we don't care about instead of tasks that are much more important to us. Understand the cost of procrastinating may not be felt until the future when the task must be completed. Completing the task immediately saves you from future repercussions that you cannot anticipate.

I previously relayed the example of people believing that at some point in the future they will be in a better mood to accomplish a task. They may believe that certain moods make them more productive and believe that they need to wait for when they are in that mood. Recognize that this is an irrational reason you are giving yourself in order to procrastinate. While your emotions can affect your work, this is only generally in the case of extremes. Slight fluctuations in mood will have no effect, so don't convince yourself that you will be in a better mood to complete the task in the future. There is no truth to this.

A more specific example of this idea that a certain mood is essential for higher productivity is the case of individuals who wait until the last moment to start a task. The student who begins to study for midterms the night before the text, or the employee who starts an project the day before it is due are two examples of this. Waiting until the last minute to start because you think you are more productive up against a deadline is nothing more than believing that your mood makes you more productive at a point in the future. Don't fall for this procrastination excuse.

An additional reason you don't want to wait until you are up against a deadline is the cognitive distortion in which you overestimate the time you have while underestimating how long it will take you to accomplish a task. If you wait, believing you work better under pressure, you may place yourself in a situation in which you have significantly underestimated the time you will need. This may cause you to rush, resulting in sub-standard work. Or, even worse, you may miss your deadline completely. Avoid backing yourself into this corner where time works against you. Remember that we often believe that we have more time than we actually do.

Another reason people often give for procrastinating is that they had forgotten about a job. Often the reason that it was forgotten is intentional, the task may be unpleasant or one that we are indifferent about. If a deadline is far into the future, it can be easy to forget about our upcoming responsibilities. Or we may believe that we will get to it closer to the deadline. Understand that this is procrastination, and that there is nothing keeping you from completing the job now.

The final cognition distortion I will address is the belief that you don't want to currently complete a job because you are not feeling well, and that you will wait until you feel better. It should be evident how this is very similar to waiting for a specific mood in order to complete a task. Understand that there is no guarantee that you will feel better, in fact, you may end up feeling worse. Granted that people suffer from real health problems that greatly impact their ability to be productive. This is not what I am referring to. Instead, I refer to procrastinators who exaggerate how they feel to shirk their responsibilities. Don't be disingenuous with yourself about how you feel in order to avoid doing something.

Many of these cognition distortions are rooted in perfectionism or in our fear. We are either waiting for the moment to be right, or we are waiting to overcome our fear to do a task we may find unpleasant. Tell yourself that the moment will never be perfect, but it will be good enough to get the job done. Or if you are dealing with fear, realize that confronting your fear and doing the job now, will mean that once you have finished you will no longer have anything to fear. In fact, you will likely feel elated. This is a much better situation to be in than living under a cloud of dread.

Now that we have explored the underlying psychological reasons behind procrastination, our attention will turn to effective methods for dealing with procrastination. By employing the appropriate methods to our life, we will be able to become happier and more productive people.

Recognize the problem

Like with any addiction or problem, the first step is always to recognize and accept that you have a problem. Since you have purchased this book, I will assume that you have identified yourself as a procrastinator, and are now taking the proper steps to remedy this.

Do not feel shamed or embarrassed, identifying and attacking your problems is a noble and brave action. Focus on your self-awareness; stopping procrastination means keeping a keen eye on your behaviors. And making the necessary corrections.

Exercise

I want you to exam your behavior and thought processes. Write down three incidents in which you procrastinated.

Refer to the previous chapter if you want to show why your reasoning was faulty.

Find the root of the problem

Why are you procrastinating? Are you a perfectionist? Is fear keeping you from accomplishing certain tasks? Be honest with yourself. Discovering the root of your procrastination is important. If you recognize the cognition distortions that you are employing, this will give you a hint at the root of your procrastination. While knowing the underlying cause is helpful, identifying your faulty reasoning so you can correct it will have greater long-term gains.

If you are a perfectionist or if fear is holding you back, I want you to take a moment and examine your thinking. Why do you have to be perfect? Does it make you more productive? Does it make you happier? My guess is the answer will be "no". Tell yourself that accomplishing something perfectly is not the goal, the goal is only accomplishing your task. Withhold judgment, jobs are either done or not done. Also, ask yourself is it true that the longer you wait, the closer you will be to perfect? Or would you have done the same job either way? Does the evidence actually support your way of thinking?

The same approach can be taken if you suffer from fear. Ask yourself what you are afraid of? Most people fear a specific outcome. Is it rational to believe that outcome is guaranteed? I may fear dying in a plane crash, so I dread getting on a plane. But what are the chances that this event actually occurs. My chances are much greater of dying in a car accident on the way to the airport, but I don't have the same dread getting into a car. By nature, fear is not rational; it often arises from the fact that we have convinced ourselves of a terrible outcome, even though that outcome may be incredibly remote. Try to look at your fear rationally; assess the likelihood of the outcomes you fear. Then ask yourself: is it really that bad? Surprisingly, our fears are often overstated; they have a tendency to shrink when we look at them rationally.

Exercise

Using the previous chapter, identify any cognitive distortions you have fallen victim to. Can you discern what is behind this? If it is fear or the desire to be perfect, look at potential outcomes. Does it really need to be perfect? Is it a situation that you should be fearful of? Write down the reasons why you believe you need to be perfect, or write down why you should be afraid. Put it away for a day, and then read it again. Do your thoughts appear logical?

Prioritize with lists

Writing down a list is very effective in helping you achieve your goals. But you need to stick with it. Many people write lists, and then don't follow them. Remember the list is to help you stop procrastinating. Once you write the list, don't convince yourself out of following the order you set.

Put the jobs in order of priority, the most important being first and the least important being last. Estimate how long you believe each task will take you. Then multiply that time by a factor of three. Set this revised time as your deadline. The extra time will take into account the possibility that you are underestimating how long each task will take you; it serves as a buffer. The benefit is that if you complete your tasks early, you now have that extra time to do things you want to.

Keep your list close at hand. You can either write it down, or like I do, keep it on a mobile device.

There are numerous to-do list apps that will simplify the process.

Exercise

Write a list in which you prioritize your tasks by level of importance. Decide how long it will take you to do each task, then multiply that number by three. Write down the time needed next to each task on your list.

Divide and conquer

There are some tasks that are so large and unwieldy that estimating how long they will take is an incredibly difficult job. To help facilitate the process, break the large job into smaller segments. These segments should be small enough that you can estimate the time each one of them will take. Make certain you add in a buffer by multiplying each estimated time by three.

If you have a specific deadline, you can now add the time estimations for each of the smaller tasks to arrive at a figure for the entire project. This is a fantastic way to estimate large projects without placing yourself in a stressful situation as the deadline approaches. In fact, this approach is used quite frequently in the software industry for large multi-team projects.

Exercise

If you have a large project on your list, particularly if you are having difficulty estimating how long it will take, break it down into smaller segments. Now evaluate how much time each task will take, keeping the added buffer in mind.

Keep distractions to a minimum

One of the biggest productivity killers in recent years for businesses has been the Internet. It becomes easier for employees to procrastinate when they have other options that are more appealing only a mouse click away. With social media and email, there is always something new happening, and it can be quite difficult not to get immersed in this flow of constant information.

There are productivity plugins that will limit your access to the Internet by allowing you to stay online for short periods of time. If possible, I also recommend shutting down your email program, and only checking it at designated times. One method that is effective is to focus on your task for the first 50 minutes in the hour. In the remaining ten minutes, you can then check your email or Facebook status.

Additionally, a work or home environment can be distracting. People talking, a television playing, and other background noise can make you lose your focus. Listening to music through headphones or using earplugs is effective in blocking out distracting noise.

Exercise

Are you being distracted? Analyze your environment and decide whether you are being distracted. If you find yourself going online to check email or surf the Internet, try to use the 50 minute rule. Browser plugins will also limit your access to the Internet. Research, install, and configure them if you need this level of restriction.

If noise is a problem, buy earplugs or bring your headphones and MP3 player in order to listen to music.

Celebrate your accomplishments

You have completed your task list; time to celebrate. Giving yourself a reward after accomplishing your goals is wonderful way to encourage yourself to leave procrastination behind. The reward can be anything, an hour of television, a movie and dinner out, or an item you want. The point is to make it something you really desire, to properly give you a sense of accomplishment.

Exercise

Schedule a reward for yourself for completing your task list. Make it good. You deserve it.

Take care of yourself

Eating right and sleeping the recommended amount by your physician is essential in helping to reduce stress and anxiety. It is much easier to tackle your task list if you are feeling energized after a good night's sleep followed by a substantial breakfast. Often poor eating habits during the day lead to your blood sugar crashing in the afternoon, leaving you feeling sluggish and tired.

Make a point of eating a balanced diet spread over at least three meals over the course of the day. Maintain a regimented sleeping schedule. Try to go to bed and wake up at approximately the same time every day. Maintaining our sleep rhythms is very important.

Exercise, put it as a high priority on your task list if you have to. This can be as simple as taking a short walk. Exercising has the wonderful effect of increasing your energy, so take advantage.

Exercise

Evaluate your eating and sleeping habits, making the necessary changes. If you are not exercising, start. It can be as simple as a thirty minute walk per day.

Learn to say no

Many of us have the tendency to want to please other people. We take on more tasks and responsibilities than we have time for, causing us to have too many things to accomplish and not enough time to do them in. If you become too overwhelmed, there is a very good chance you will procrastinate rather than tackle your enormous list.

Learning to say no to task of low importance is key. When someone asks you to do something, look at what they are asking objectively. Is this task a high priority to you? What is the opportunity cost to you? Remember that your time is extremely valuable, it cannot be replaced. Time you spend on this task could be spent elsewhere. Unless it is a close family member, the most time I'm willing to spend on a task for someone is ten minutes. If I don't think I can accomplish it in ten minutes (after adding in my buffer), I will apologize and tell the person that I can't do it. Most people understand, they realize that we all lead busy lives. And if they don't, it is only further justification that I made the right decision.

Exercise

Look at your task list. Are there low priority jobs on it that you agreed to do for other people? If so, remove them from your list and let the person know, unless you believe you can accomplish it in a very short timeframe.

Be proactive in obtaining the information you need

During our examination of cognition distortions, we talked about procrastinating because we lack specific information about how to proceed or what our ultimate goal was. The way to avoid this problem is to always ask questions immediately on being given the task. Make certain you understand what your deliverables will be as well as the best way to proceed. There is no harm in asking and getting the answer. It will save you both time and aggravation.

With the advent of cellphones and email, people are generally accessible within a few hours. If the person you need to ask is not available, try to ask someone who has completed a similar task. Asking questions is not only an effective method for curtailing procrastination, it also has a generally positive affect on your life. We live in a society where the majority of people ask too few questions.

Exercise

Examine your task list. Is there a task that you have questions about? If so, contact the person who can answer your questions immediately. Even if it is late, send them an email. Don't wait, act on your questions right now.

Get into the habit

Procrastination is a bad habit, emphasis on habit. Habits need to be broken, and the best way to accomplish this is by replacing them with a new habit. If you have taken the suggested action to this point, you have already started on your way to replacing your habit to procrastinate. But it is only the start. Generally, it is believed that if a person can change their behavior for twenty-one days that change will become permanent.

Exercise

Find a calendar and mark off twenty-one days from today. Your goal is to keep up on doing your task list daily for the twenty-one days. Be aware that you will have to fight to keep procrastination from coming back in. Replacing old habits can be difficult, which means you need to remain vigilant of any back-sliding.

Make tasks relevant to you

Many of the jobs we do are done despite us being indifferent to the task or not enjoying it. The easiest way to combat this is to look at the task and accentuate a positive aspect of it. If you can find a good reason for doing something, it will make accomplishing it much more attractive to you. Think outside the box for reasons if you have to. Maybe completing a task will open up a new opportunity in your life, or allow you to connect with different people. Accomplishing it may give you the opportunity to make new friends.

There are a variety of reasons why a task should be completed. You need to find the one that holds the most appeal to you.

Exercise

Take a moment to examine your list. Are there any jobs you do not enjoy to do? Are there any tasks you feel indifferent about? If so, think of a good reason, one that appeals to you, of what completing the task could mean for you. Try to find a reason that makes you want to tackle the job.

Conclusion

I hope that you have found this journey helpful. If you have participated in the recommended exercises along the way, you should be commended. You have clearly decided you want to change, and that is a huge first step to becoming a more productive person.

Procrastination is not something you need to suffer with, the answers are all right here in this guide. Understand that procrastination can have deep psychological roots, causes that take time and effort to overcome. The best way to accomplish this is to face it head on. If you are a perfectionist, try completing a task even though you may not feel it is perfect, or up to your usual standards. If fear is holding you back, stand up to it by imagining the worst outcome, and then honestly evaluating how likely that outcome will come to be.

Humans suffer from many irrational thoughts, convinced of the truth of an idea even though the evidence suggests the opposite. Recognizing these irrational thoughts is the first step in dispelling them. Once you realize you are being illogical, the thought fails to hold any power over you anymore. Never take anything for granted, continuously question your thoughts, assessing them for validity. This isn't only the key to stopping procrastination, it also leads to a life that is happier and more productive.

I wish you all the success in your journey.

WAIT! Before You Leave…

Download the #1 Bestseller from Gamma Mouse Media for FREE! Hurry this offer won't last as it is for a limited time only. Reserve your free copy today at http://gammamouse.com.

Made in the USA
Lexington, KY
15 September 2015